DMSO

Your Natural Defense Against Pain and Inflammation. A Practical Guide to Natural Healing with Dimethyl Sulfoxide for Chronic Pain, Inflammation, and Total Body Wellness

Rachel Haines

Contents

Introduction	v
1. DMSO Basics – What It Is and Why It Works	1
2. Getting Started – DMSO Application 101	11
3. Targeting Pain with DMSO	21
4. Healing Skin Conditions Naturally with DMSO	29
5. Internal Uses of DMSO and Controversies	37
6. Using DMSO for Athletic Performance	45
7. Beyond Pain – DMSO for Everyday Wellness	51
8. Advanced Tips and FAQs for Mastering DMSO Use	61
Epilogue	69
DMSO Usage Checklist	73
Safe Mixing, Storing, and Application	77

Introduction

Imagine finding relief in a single, simple compound that's been used for decades yet remains largely under the radar. That's the promise of DMSO, or Dimethyl Sulfoxide—a natural remedy, derived originally from wood pulp, that has found its way into the hands of individuals desperate for alternatives to conventional painkillers and anti-inflammatory medications. DMSO has earned a quiet but devoted following among those who've experienced firsthand its ability to relieve pain, soothe inflammation, and promote healing at the cellular level.

Dr. Stanley Jacob, often called the father of DMSO research, famously said, "In my experience, DMSO is the closest thing to a panacea that I've seen." Such a bold statement from a respected medical professional is rare, and it captures the enthusiasm many feel about DMSO's potential. But what exactly is DMSO, and why has it captivated so many? To understand its appeal, we need to look at its journey from industrial byproduct to potent healing solution.

The History of DMSO: From Wood Pulp to Modern Medicine

DMSO's story begins in the 19th century, where it was first discovered as a byproduct of the wood processing industry. In those early days, it was merely a curious, colorless liquid with a strong, slightly garlicky odor, used primarily as a solvent in laboratory settings. But DMSO didn't stay unnoticed for long. Researchers observed something unusual about it: unlike other solvents, DMSO could slip effortlessly through cell membranes. Even more intriguing, it could carry other substances with it, acting as a kind of molecular transport system. This unique ability set DMSO apart and piqued scientific curiosity, signaling that it might have potential beyond its industrial applications.

It wasn't until the 1960s, however, that DMSO began to be explored as a health-promoting substance. Dr. Stanley Jacob, a surgeon and researcher at the Oregon Health & Science University, spearheaded pioneering studies into DMSO's properties. Fascinated by its potential, Dr. Jacob discovered that DMSO had remarkable anti-inflammatory and analgesic effects. These findings opened the door to a new realm of possibility, hinting that DMSO could be used to relieve pain, reduce inflammation, and even support healing in a way that traditional

Introduction

pain relievers could not. Dr. Jacob's work with DMSO attracted international attention and generated a groundswell of enthusiasm among scientists and healthcare practitioners. DMSO seemed poised to become a groundbreaking treatment in modern medicine.

Yet, DMSO's journey was far from smooth. Despite its promising benefits, it faced resistance and regulatory hurdles. While countries like Russia embraced it widely, using it to treat pain, inflammation, sports injuries, and even as a supportive therapy in certain chronic conditions, other regions were more cautious. In the United States, for instance, DMSO encountered considerable pushback from regulatory bodies. The FDA limited its approval to very specific medical applications, such as treating interstitial cystitis, a painful bladder condition, while dismissing its broader therapeutic potential. Despite mounting evidence of its benefits, mainstream acceptance remained elusive, and DMSO became one of medicine's more controversial substances.

For years, its benefits went largely unnoticed by the general public. But DMSO found a loyal following in niche communities—athletes, alternative health practitioners, and individuals seeking natural approaches to health and wellness. Many who had tried DMSO spoke of its transformative effects, often sharing personal stories of pain relief and improved mobility that defied the limitations of conventional treatments. This underground reputation as a "miracle" compound kept DMSO relevant, if somewhat hidden from mainstream view.

Introduction

In recent years, however, DMSO has seen a resurgence. As more people explore alternatives to synthetic drugs and embrace natural, holistic health practices, DMSO's unique properties have brought it back into the spotlight. Its ability to address pain and inflammation, combined with its minimal side effects when used correctly, appeals to individuals seeking safer, more effective ways to support their health. For a substance that began as a humble byproduct, DMSO's journey has been nothing short of remarkable, spanning decades of scientific exploration, regulatory battles, and renewed interest as people search for options outside of conventional medicine.

Today, DMSO is a symbol of the growing movement toward natural wellness. It represents a shift in health perspectives, a return to simpler, evidence-backed solutions that work with the body instead of against it. As research continues and more people discover its benefits, DMSO may well cement its place as a trusted, versatile ally in the pursuit of health and healing. Its history, from a little-known solvent to a game-changing therapeutic tool, is a testament to the power of scientific curiosity and the timeless appeal of nature's remedies.

Why People Turn to DMSO

For anyone who's tried—and failed—to find lasting relief from persistent pain or relentless inflammation, the appeal of DMSO is immediate and understandable. Conventional treatments often come with a catch: they

Introduction

mask symptoms without addressing the root cause, or they bring with them a list of side effects that can feel as exhausting as the condition itself. DMSO offers a refreshing alternative. Unlike many pharmaceuticals, it doesn't just dull the senses or put a temporary bandage over the pain. Instead, it works directly on the problem, targeting inflammation at the source and supporting cellular repair in the process. For those who feel they've tried everything else, DMSO can feel like a breath of fresh air—a solution that finally makes sense and works with the body rather than overriding its natural processes.

People are increasingly drawn to natural remedies, seeking alternatives that don't carry the risks or dependency of traditional medications. This shift is significant. A survey by the American Association of Naturopathic Physicians found that nearly 60% of people in the U.S. have turned to some form of complementary medicine, a figure that speaks volumes about the growing dissatisfaction with conventional treatments. Among those surveyed, more than a third cited a strong preference for natural, non-invasive solutions—a desire to feel well without the "trade-offs" that so often come with pharmaceuticals. In this landscape, DMSO fits perfectly. It's a natural compound with the power to relieve pain, reduce inflammation, and restore mobility, without the baggage of unwanted side effects or the fear of long-term dependency.

The experiences of DMSO users echo these sentiments. Many report improvements not only in pain relief

Introduction

but in mobility, flexibility, and overall well-being. Within just a few applications, users commonly feel a marked difference, often describing the relief as transformative. In an era where people are exhausted by endless pill regimens, DMSO offers hope in its simplicity, effectiveness, and natural origins. It's more than just a remedy; it's a shift toward a holistic, empowering approach to health that resonates with a new generation of health-conscious individuals looking for genuine, sustainable solutions.

Setting Expectations for This Book

This book is crafted as a comprehensive guide to help you safely and effectively bring DMSO into your wellness routine. Whether your goal is to manage chronic pain, reduce persistent inflammation, or simply explore a natural alternative for health maintenance, DMSO has the potential to become a valuable addition to your approach. But like any powerful tool, using DMSO correctly is essential. Each chapter is designed to equip you with clear, actionable knowledge—everything from choosing the right type and concentration of DMSO to mastering safe, effective application methods. With the right information, you'll be empowered to maximize DMSO's benefits in a way that supports your unique health goals.

You'll find step-by-step guidance, practical tips, and answers to the most common questions surrounding DMSO use. For those who are entirely new to DMSO, this book serves as an introduction to what it is, how it

Introduction

works, and why so many people have found it worth adding to their daily health regimen. Each section builds a strong foundation, explaining DMSO's mechanisms in accessible terms, so you'll feel confident in every step of your journey. For readers already familiar with DMSO, we've included advanced techniques and insights—ways to combine it with other natural remedies, adapt it to specific needs, and take your results to the next level.

Ultimately, this book is about giving you a practical toolkit to unlock DMSO's potential. By the end, you'll understand why DMSO is often considered a "secret weapon" against pain and inflammation and see how it can become a dependable, versatile solution in your own wellness routine. So whether you're here to find immediate relief or seeking a long-term, holistic approach to health, this guide will be your trusted resource on every step of the journey.

40

Chapter 1

DMSO Basics – What It Is and Why It Works

"DMSO is a simple molecule with powerful potential."
— Dr. Stanley Jacob, Father of DMSO Research

DMSO, or Dimethyl Sulfoxide, might seem unassuming at first glance, but it holds surprising power. This colorless, odorless liquid, born from the wood pulp industry, is more than just a chemical compound; it's a natural remedy that's intrigued scientists, doctors, and those seeking relief from pain and inflammation for decades. Often described as a "miracle" molecule, DMSO has the ability to penetrate deeply into tissues, reaching places that many traditional treatments struggle to impact.

Originally discovered in the 19th century as a byproduct of wood processing, DMSO was initially used as an industrial solvent, prized for its ability to dissolve other compounds effortlessly. Yet it wasn't until the 1960s that researchers began to consider its potential therapeutic applications. Dr. Stanley Jacob, a pioneer in DMSO research, was instrumental in transforming this simple molecule into a groundbreaking treatment option. As he explored its effects, he noted DMSO's remarkable ability to relieve pain and reduce inflammation, and he quickly realized that this solvent had become something much more valuable—a medical tool with profound implications.

1.1 What Is DMSO?

DMSO, or Dimethyl Sulfoxide, stands out in the world of natural health solutions due to its unique structure and impressive abilities. This small molecule has an extraordinary talent: it can penetrate cell membranes with remarkable ease. Unlike larger compounds that are blocked by the body's natural barriers, DMSO slips through effortlessly, reaching areas that many treatments cannot. This deep permeability is the key to DMSO's effectiveness; by moving through barriers that would typically stop other substances, it can deliver its therapeutic effects exactly where they're needed—deep into joints, muscles, and even nerve tissues.

This exceptional ability sets DMSO apart from mainstream pain relief options. While most over-the-counter painkillers only mask pain for a few hours, DMSO goes beyond surface-level relief. It doesn't just dull the sensation—it targets the root cause of pain by addressing inflammation and supporting cellular repair. DMSO works with the body's own processes to facilitate true healing, not just temporary comfort. And because DMSO is derived from a natural process—it was first found as a byproduct of wood pulp processing—it appeals to those looking for more natural alternatives. Many people are drawn to DMSO as a way to avoid the synthetic chemicals and potential side effects common with pharmaceuticals.

For those who are tired of the conventional "take two and wait" approach, DMSO offers something refreshingly different. It brings relief without the numbing side effects that often accompany painkillers, and without the risks associated with prolonged pharmaceutical use. DMSO's appeal lies in its simplicity and effectiveness, offering people a natural, potent solution that targets pain and inflammation at the source, supporting their journey to real, sustainable healing.

1.2 How DMSO Works at the Cellular Level

To truly grasp why DMSO is so effective, we need to look at its function inside the body at a microscopic level. Within the cells, DMSO acts as a potent anti-inflammatory agent, targeting one of the primary culprits of chronic pain: inflammation. Normally, inflammation is part of the body's natural response to injury, signaling immune cells to help repair damaged tissues. But when inflammation becomes prolonged or excessive, it can cause more harm than good, leading to ongoing discomfort and stiffness. DMSO works by directly reducing this inflammation, relieving the pressure and sensitivity around nerve endings, which in turn alleviates pain. It doesn't merely mask pain; it addresses the root issue, helping to restore balance and comfort to affected tissues.

But DMSO's capabilities don't stop at reducing inflammation. It also boasts powerful antioxidant properties, which help combat oxidative stress—a damaging process linked to aging, cell deterioration, and numerous chronic diseases. Oxidative stress occurs when free radicals, or unstable molecules, start to damage healthy cells, accelerating cellular wear and tear. By neutralizing these free radicals, DMSO protects cells and promotes healthier, more resilient tissues. Dr. Stanley Jacob, a pioneer in DMSO research, once noted, "It's almost as if DMSO rejuvenates the tissue," underscoring its potential not just for managing symptoms but for enhancing overall cellular health.

So, what sets DMSO apart from traditional treatments? One reason is that DMSO doesn't merely cover up symptoms. Instead, it aligns with the body's own healing processes, supporting and amplifying them. Acting almost as a cellular guide, DMSO facilitates the delivery of other beneficial compounds to targeted areas, enhancing their effectiveness. This "carrier" quality is one of its most valuable traits, as it allows users to combine DMSO with other treatments, such as herbal extracts or topical creams, to create a synergistic effect. By helping these compounds penetrate deeply into tissues, DMSO maximizes their therapeutic potential, making it an incredibly versatile tool in natural health.

1.3 DMSO's Healing Benefits Beyond Pain Relief

While DMSO is primarily known for its pain-relieving properties, its benefits extend beyond that. For those struggling with joint pain, DMSO has become a lifeline. Its ability to penetrate deep into joint tissues provides targeted relief for arthritis and related conditions. Individuals using DMSO for joint pain often report improvements in mobility and reduced stiffness, describing it as a sense of "freedom" that they hadn't felt in years.

Beyond joint pain, DMSO offers benefits for skin health. People dealing with acne, minor cuts, and even scars have found that DMSO aids in the healing process. Applied topically, it reduces redness and helps wounds close up more quickly. For individuals with chronic skin conditions like eczema or psoriasis, DMSO has shown potential as a soothing agent, reducing inflammation and calming irritated skin.

There's even evidence suggesting that DMSO can benefit systemic conditions such as neuropathy, a nerve-related issue that causes discomfort and numbness. Some users have reported that consistent use of DMSO reduces their symptoms, though it's essential to approach these claims with caution until more research can substantiate them. Still, the personal stories surrounding DMSO's effectiveness are hard to ignore.

1.4 Safety Precautions and Potential Side Effects

Like any powerful remedy, DMSO must be used responsibly. While generally considered safe, there are some side effects that users should be aware of, the most common being a garlic-like odor that can linger on the skin after application. This occurs because DMSO contains sulfur, which the body metabolizes in a way that produces this distinctive smell. For some, it's a minor inconvenience; for others, it can be bothersome, so it's best to start with a small application to see how your body reacts.

Purity is another important consideration. Not all DMSO products are created equal, and it's crucial to select a high-purity DMSO that's intended for human use. Products with a purity of 99% or higher are generally recommended, as impurities can introduce unnecessary risks. Additionally, DMSO comes in different concentrations, typically diluted with water or aloe vera, and choosing the right concentration can make a difference in both safety and effectiveness. Experts advise beginning with a lower concentration and gradually increasing if your body responds well.

Finally, testing a small area before a full application is always wise, particularly if you have sensitive skin. DMSO is a potent substance, and a patch test can prevent unwanted reactions. This gradual approach allows you to assess how your skin and body handle DMSO, setting the stage for safer, more informed use.

1.5 Choosing the Right DMSO for You

Selecting the right form of DMSO is key to maximizing its benefits. Available in liquid, gel, and cream forms, each type offers unique advantages depending on your needs. Liquids are ideal for deep, penetrating applications and can be diluted to different strengths, while gels are often preferred for joint and muscle applications where the gel's consistency makes it easier to control. Creams, on the other hand, are typically combined with soothing ingredients like aloe vera, making them gentler and a better choice for sensitive areas or daily use.

Labels are another critical aspect to consider. Not all DMSO products are labeled for human use, and it's essential to look for reputable brands that clearly state their DMSO is pharmaceutical grade. Reading the label carefully will help you avoid products intended for industrial or laboratory use, which may contain impurities unsuitable for skin application.

Where to buy DMSO can also make a difference in quality. Many health stores and online retailers offer

DMSO, but it's wise to stick to trusted suppliers that have positive customer feedback and transparent sourcing practices. DMSO's effectiveness is directly tied to its purity, so choosing the right product is an important first step in your journey toward relief.

Chapter 2

Getting Started – DMSO Application 101

"DMSO's biggest strength lies in its versatility—learn how to harness it."

Now that you understand DMSO's impressive potential, it's time to focus on getting started with its application. Applying DMSO is simple, but getting the most out of it requires attention to a few key details, from skin preparation to dilution ratios to the tools you'll use. With the right approach, DMSO can be an incredibly effective, safe addition to your health routine. This chapter will walk you through each step, ensuring you feel confident, informed, and prepared to begin using DMSO effectively.

2.1 Preparing Your Skin for Application

DMSO's unique ability to penetrate the skin deeply is one of its greatest advantages. But this also means that it's crucial to apply DMSO on clean skin. Any contaminants —like lotions, oils, or even microscopic particles—can be carried into the skin along with the DMSO, which could cause irritation or reduce effectiveness.

Before application, clean the skin thoroughly with a gentle, fragrance-free soap, and rinse with water. Avoid using lotions or oils beforehand, as these can interfere with DMSO's absorption. For individuals with sensitive skin or applying DMSO to areas prone to irritation, doing a quick patch test on a small spot is wise. Apply a diluted version of DMSO to a small area, wait, and check for any adverse reactions. This simple precaution can save you from discomfort later on.

2.2 How to Measure and Dilute DMSO Safely

Diluting DMSO is a crucial step, especially for first-time users or those applying it to more sensitive areas of the body. While DMSO's full strength can be incredibly effective, it's also highly potent, and undiluted use may cause irritation or discomfort. Understanding proper dilution ratios not only ensures safety but also allows you to tailor the application to your specific needs.

For beginners, it's generally recommended to start with a 70% DMSO to 30% water solution. This dilution strikes a balance between potency and safety, offering effective results without overwhelming the skin. If this concentration feels too strong—causing tingling or mild irritation—you can easily adjust by increasing the water content. Some users find that starting with a 50% solution works better for their comfort, particularly when applying DMSO to delicate areas like the neck, wrists, or behind the knees.

The choice of mixing medium plays a significant role in how DMSO interacts with your skin. While distilled water is the simplest and most commonly used option, it's not the only one. Aloe vera gel is a popular alternative, offering a soothing base that helps mitigate the initial tingling sensation some people experience when first using DMSO. The cooling, anti-inflammatory properties of aloe vera complement DMSO's effects, making it an excellent choice for those with sensitive skin or those applying DMSO to areas prone to irritation. Another advantage of aloe vera is its gel-like consistency, which makes application more controlled and less likely to drip.

When preparing your solution, precision is key. Use a clean, graduated dropper or measuring cup to ensure accurate ratios. For example, to create a 70% solution, combine 7 parts DMSO with 3 parts distilled water or aloe vera gel. Always mix in a glass container, as DMSO can react with certain plastics, potentially contaminating the solution.

It's also important to note that dilution isn't a one-size-fits-all process. Your skin's reaction to DMSO can vary depending on the application area, your personal sensitivity, and even your hydration levels. Start with a lower concentration, especially if you're new to DMSO, and gradually increase as your skin becomes accustomed to it. Observing how your body responds over the first few applications will help you find the right balance between effectiveness and comfort.

2.3 Step-by-Step Guide to Applying DMSO

Once you've prepared your diluted solution and cleaned the area of skin where you plan to apply it, you're ready to begin. Proper application is key to maximizing DMSO's benefits while minimizing the risk of irritation or contamination. Follow these steps to ensure a safe and effective experience.

First, choose an applicator that suits your needs. A cotton ball or a clean, soft cloth works well for most applications, providing an even spread without over-saturating the skin. If you're working with smaller areas or precise spots, a cotton swab can offer better control. For those using higher concentrations of DMSO or who have particularly sensitive skin, wearing gloves is highly recommended. Latex or nitrile gloves are ideal, as they prevent DMSO from absorbing into your hands and carrying any contaminants from your skin into the treated area. Remember, DMSO's powerful ability to penetrate means it can transport impurities as well, so cleanliness is crucial at every step.

When applying DMSO, gently dab or smooth the solution onto the target area. There's no need to rub it in vigorously—DMSO naturally penetrates the skin within seconds, carrying its therapeutic effects deep into tissues. Over-application won't increase its effectiveness and may only lead to irritation. Aim for a light, even layer that fully covers the area of concern.

After application, allow the area to air dry. This typically takes a few minutes, depending on the concentration and the amount applied. During this time, avoid touching the treated skin to prevent accidental transfer of DMSO to other areas, especially sensitive regions like the face or eyes. Similarly, ensure that clothing or bedding doesn't come into contact with the area until it's fully absorbed.

Some users may experience a mild tingling or warming sensation shortly after application, particularly if they're new to DMSO. This is a common reaction and usually subsides within a few minutes. However, if you notice persistent discomfort, redness, or itching, it's a sign that your skin may need a gentler approach. In such cases, consider diluting your solution further for future applications. For example, if you started with a 70% solution, try reducing it to 50% to see if it improves your comfort level.

2.4 Combining DMSO with Other Natural Remedies

One of DMSO's most impressive features is its ability to act as a transdermal carrier, allowing other substances to penetrate the skin and reach deeper tissues with greater efficiency. This unique property opens up a world of possibilities for enhancing the effectiveness of natural remedies by combining them with DMSO. Whether you're seeking pain relief, improved skin health, or targeted recovery after physical exertion, DMSO can amplify the benefits of other treatments, making it a powerful tool in your wellness arsenal.

For muscle cramps or tension, many users pair DMSO with magnesium oil. Magnesium is known for its ability to relax muscles and reduce cramping, but when combined with DMSO, its absorption improves significantly, delivering faster and more pronounced relief. Similarly, vitamin C, a potent antioxidant, can be used alongside DMSO to combat oxidative stress and promote cellular repair. By carrying vitamin C deeper into the tissues, DMSO may enhance its ability to neutralize free radicals and support the body's natural healing processes.

Customizing DMSO blends allows you to tailor treatments to your specific needs. For instance, if you're dealing with both joint pain and sensitive skin, you might combine DMSO with aloe vera gel for a soothing, anti-inflammatory application. Aloe vera not only provides hydration and cooling relief but also helps reduce the tingling sensation that DMSO can sometimes cause, especially for new users. Adding a few drops of lavender essential oil to this blend creates a calming, spa-like experience, ideal for winding down after a stressful day or a vigorous workout.

However, it's essential to approach these combinations with care. DMSO's ability to enhance absorption means that any compound it carries will enter your system more quickly and directly. This is a double-edged sword; while it amplifies the benefits of safe, natural ingredients, it can also increase the risk of irritation or unwanted side effects if the wrong substances are used. To avoid this, always start with a low concentration of DMSO when trying new mixtures and apply a small amount to a test area on your skin. Monitor for any signs of irritation, such as redness, itching, or discomfort, before proceeding with full applications.

When creating custom blends, stick to ingredients that are known to be skin-safe and compatible with your health goals. Avoid mixing DMSO with products containing synthetic chemicals, fragrances, or alcohol, as these can cause irritation or other adverse effects. By thoughtfully combining DMSO with complementary remedies, you can harness its full potential to support your body in a safe and effective way. The result is a personalized, holistic approach to health that addresses multiple concerns at once, offering a more dynamic and satisfying wellness experience.

2.5 Creating a Routine That Works for You

With DMSO, consistency is key, but overuse can lead to diminishing returns or even mild skin irritation. Many users find that applying DMSO once or twice a day works well for chronic pain or persistent inflammation, while others find relief with less frequent applications. Track your results and be patient; like any natural remedy, DMSO works best as part of a consistent, long-term approach.

It can also be helpful to keep a simple log of your applications, noting any changes you experience. This could be as basic as jotting down dates, times, and any observed effects, or using a dedicated app if that's your style. Adjust your frequency as you go; some people find they need less over time, while others prefer to maintain a regular routine.

Chapter 3

Targeting Pain with DMSO

For anyone who has suffered from chronic pain, the idea of waking up free from it can feel like an unreachable dream. Pain can be isolating, relentless, and exhausting. Traditional medications may offer temporary relief, but the need to continuously mask pain often leads to frustration and a growing sense of helplessness. This is where DMSO offers something genuinely different. Unlike conventional painkillers, which simply block pain signals, DMSO works deeper, addressing the roots of pain, reducing inflammation, and promoting real healing in the tissues.

In this chapter, we'll explore how DMSO targets various types of pain—from joint pain to nerve discomfort—and how you can apply it to find relief that's lasting and meaningful.

. . .

3.1 Understanding Pain Types and Their Causes

Pain is a complex and deeply personal experience, varying widely not just in intensity but in its origin and nature. To harness DMSO's full potential, it's crucial to understand the different types of pain and their underlying causes. Broadly speaking, pain can be classified into two main categories: acute and chronic. Each type presents unique challenges and requires a tailored approach for effective management.

Acute pain is immediate and often sharp, typically arising from a specific injury, surgery, or sudden illness. It serves as a warning signal, alerting the body to potential harm. This type of pain is generally short-lived, subsiding as the underlying issue heals. For example, the searing pain from a sprained ankle or a surgical incision is acute—it's intense but temporary, often diminishing as tissues repair themselves over days or weeks. Acute pain, though uncomfortable, usually responds well to conventional treatments like over-the-counter painkillers or ice packs.

Chronic pain, however, is an entirely different beast. It lingers for months, sometimes years, often persisting long after the initial injury or illness has resolved. Unlike acute pain, which has a clear beginning and end, chronic pain can feel endless, wearing down both the body and the spirit. Conditions like arthritis, fibromyalgia, or nerve damage frequently involve chronic pain, which is often accompanied by inflammation. This inflammation not only causes discomfort but can also damage surrounding tissues over time, creating a vicious cycle that's difficult to break.

Traditional pain management strategies, such as prescription medications, often fall short in addressing chronic pain. These treatments tend to focus on masking the sensation of pain rather than tackling its root causes. This is where DMSO stands out.

Unlike typical pain relievers, which work superficially, DMSO penetrates deeply into tissues, targeting the cellular mechanisms behind pain. Its anti-inflammatory properties help reduce swelling and pressure on nerves, while its antioxidant effects combat oxidative stress—a key contributor to long-term tissue damage and pain persistence.

What makes DMSO particularly effective is its ability to address pain at the source. For chronic pain sufferers, this can be a game-changer. Instead of simply dulling the sensation for a few hours, DMSO works to resolve the underlying issues contributing to pain, such as inflammation and cellular damage. This means that with regular use, many people experience not only relief but also improved mobility and a gradual reduction in pain severity over time.

3.2 DMSO for Joint Pain Relief

Joint pain is one of the most common and challenging types of chronic pain, affecting millions of people who struggle with arthritis, rheumatic conditions, or injuries that don't seem to heal. For those dealing with joint pain, applying DMSO can be transformative. DMSO is especially effective for arthritis because it reduces the inflammation within the joints, relieving the swelling and stiffness that make movement difficult and painful.

For example, someone with arthritis in their knees might apply DMSO directly to the joint, allowing it to penetrate deep into the tissue. This localized treatment can reduce inflammation and improve joint mobility, making daily activities less painful. DMSO also works well on smaller joints, like those in the wrists or fingers, where rheumatic pain often strikes. For safe application, it's best to start with a diluted DMSO solution and observe how your body responds before increasing the concentration. Many find that regular, careful application helps maintain flexibility and reduces the flare-ups that are so common with joint pain.

3.3 Muscle Pain and DMSO's Role

Muscle pain, whether from strain, exercise, or tension, can be surprisingly debilitating. Athletes, in particular, are drawn to DMSO because it aids recovery and reduces muscle soreness after intense workouts. Applied to the affected muscles, DMSO helps clear out lactic acid buildup, one of the primary contributors to post-exercise soreness. This speeds up recovery time, allowing athletes to maintain a consistent training schedule without being sidelined by muscle fatigue.

For muscle recovery, DMSO can be applied both before and after workouts. Pre-exercise application helps prepare muscles for strain, while post-exercise use aids in faster recovery. Those who regularly engage in physical activity find that DMSO offers a natural way to manage the wear and tear that comes with training. For anyone seeking faster recovery from muscle strain or general fatigue, a light application of DMSO on sore areas followed by gentle stretching can be incredibly effective in relaxing and restoring muscles.

3.4 Nerve Pain Relief with DMSO

Nerve pain, or neuropathic pain, is another area where DMSO has shown great promise. Unlike pain in muscles or joints, nerve pain often feels like sharp, shooting sensations or persistent tingling and numbness. For people dealing with sciatica or lower back issues, finding relief can be challenging because the pain originates from nerve irritation, not tissue inflammation alone. However, DMSO's penetrating properties allow it to reach nerve tissues, where it can reduce the inflammation that presses on the nerves and creates pain.

When using DMSO for nerve pain, particularly in sensitive areas like the lower back, it's important to use a gentle application method and start with a lower concentration. Some users combine DMSO with gentle stretching exercises or complementary nerve treatments, finding that this combination enhances relief. As DMSO works to alleviate the underlying inflammation, regular use can lead to a noticeable reduction in nerve pain frequency and intensity, making it easier to manage daily activities without interruption.

3.5 Headaches and Migraines: DMSO's Surprising Benefits

One of the more surprising benefits of DMSO is its potential to relieve headaches and migraines. For tension headaches, which are often caused by tight muscles in the neck and scalp, DMSO can be applied topically to these areas. This helps relax the muscles and reduce the pressure that triggers headache pain. Some users have also found that small, diluted applications around the temples or back of the neck help reduce the intensity of migraines when they start.

It's worth noting that while DMSO can provide relief, it's essential to be cautious with applications around the head and neck. Small-scale applications, using a low concentration, are recommended. Some people find that using DMSO at the first sign of a headache can prevent it from escalating into a full-blown migraine, making it an invaluable tool for anyone who frequently deals with these types of pain.

Chapter 4

Healing Skin Conditions Naturally with DMSO

DMSO's benefits aren't limited to relieving pain—it also offers promising results for skin health. For centuries, people have sought remedies to help clear breakouts, reduce scarring, soothe chronic skin conditions, and even slow the signs of aging. DMSO, with its unique properties, provides a natural, versatile option for addressing these concerns. Its deep penetration and anti-inflammatory capabilities make it a valuable tool for promoting healthier, clearer skin.

In this chapter, we'll explore how DMSO can help with acne, scars, eczema, wounds, and aging, offering practical tips and safe techniques for each type of skin concern.

4.1 DMSO for Acne and Breakouts

Acne can be a persistent, frustrating issue, often driven by bacteria, inflammation, and clogged pores. DMSO's antibacterial and anti-inflammatory properties make it especially effective for managing breakouts. As it penetrates deeply into the skin, DMSO can help reduce redness and swelling around blemishes, creating a calming effect that can ease the intensity of breakouts.

However, due to its strength, it's important to apply DMSO carefully to avoid irritation, especially on sensitive or already inflamed skin. Many users find that a low concentration, around 30-50%, is ideal for acne-prone areas, as this is less likely to cause a strong reaction. When applying DMSO to the skin, consider pairing it with natural oils, such as jojoba or tea tree oil, which can further balance and soothe skin without clogging pores. This combination provides an antibacterial and moisturizing effect, helping to clear and calm the skin without overdrying.

4.2 Scar Reduction with DMSO

DMSO's ability to soften and smooth skin can also aid in reducing the appearance of scars. Whether dealing with stretch marks, surgical scars, or marks left from previous injuries, DMSO can help break down the fibrous tissue that causes scars to feel rough or raised. For older scars, this softening effect may take time, but with consistent application, many users report noticeable improvements in texture and color.

Applying DMSO directly to scars is relatively simple. A gel form is often preferred, as it adheres better to the skin and is easy to target on specific areas. While complete removal of scars is unlikely, users can expect a softening and fading of scar tissue over time, giving skin a smoother, more even appearance. For deeper scars, patience is key, and setting realistic expectations is essential—while DMSO can be transformative, it works gradually, especially on older, established scars.

4.3 Eczema and Psoriasis Relief

For those suffering from chronic conditions like eczema and psoriasis, flare-ups can be both physically and emotionally taxing. These conditions often cause redness, itchiness, and irritation, sometimes making even basic activities uncomfortable. DMSO offers a gentle yet effective way to help manage these symptoms by reducing inflammation and soothing the skin.

When creating a DMSO routine for eczema or psoriasis, consistency is crucial. Many find that applying a diluted DMSO solution—often combined with soothing ingredients like aloe vera—on a daily basis provides the best results. This mixture can be applied to affected areas, helping to calm inflamed skin and reduce itchiness. Users who combine DMSO with other natural remedies, such as chamomile or calendula, report enhanced relief, as these botanicals have additional anti-inflammatory and skin-soothing properties.

4.4 Minor Cuts, Burns, and Wounds

DMSO's role in wound healing is one of its lesser-known benefits but can be incredibly useful in managing minor skin injuries. Applied to small cuts, scrapes, or even minor burns, DMSO supports the skin's natural healing process by reducing inflammation and increasing circulation to the area. This can lead to faster healing with less risk of scarring.

When applying DMSO to fresh wounds, it's best to dilute it, as high concentrations can cause irritation on open skin. Starting with a 30-50% solution and applying it with a cotton swab is often ideal for sensitive or recently damaged areas. DMSO can also be combined with a natural antiseptic, like diluted tea tree oil, to keep the wound clean and promote a more seamless recovery. Many users find that with regular application, their cuts and scrapes heal without the thick, fibrous scarring that can sometimes occur with untreated wounds.

4.5 Anti-Aging Benefits of DMSO

One of the most intriguing applications of DMSO is its potential to slow the visible signs of aging and rejuvenate the skin. As we age, our skin undergoes a gradual loss of elasticity, moisture, and firmness, leading to the development of fine lines, wrinkles, and uneven texture. This process is largely driven by a combination of reduced collagen production, environmental damage, and oxidative stress. DMSO, with its unique ability to penetrate deeply into the skin, offers a natural solution that works at the cellular level to combat these effects, promoting healthier, more youthful-looking skin from the inside out.

What sets DMSO apart from conventional anti-aging treatments is its capacity to enhance cellular health. By reducing inflammation and oxidative stress—two major contributors to skin aging—DMSO helps preserve the integrity of skin cells and encourages their regeneration. Its deep-penetrating action ensures that these benefits reach beyond the surface, targeting the very structures that support skin elasticity and firmness. Over time, this can result in a noticeable improvement in skin texture, tone, and overall appearance.

For those looking to incorporate DMSO into their anti-aging routine, consistency is crucial. A common approach is to mix a small amount of DMSO with a hydrating serum or a few drops of vitamin C, both of which are well-known for their skin-nourishing properties. Vitamin C, in particular, boosts collagen production and provides antioxidant protection, complementing DMSO's ability to neutralize free radicals. When applied weekly, this combination can help enhance the skin's natural glow, reduce the appearance of fine lines, and create a smoother, firmer texture. However, care should be taken to avoid the delicate eye area and other sensitive spots, as these regions may react more strongly to DMSO.

For optimal results, it's important to integrate DMSO

into a broader skincare regimen that includes hydration, sun protection, and a balanced diet rich in skin-friendly nutrients. Unlike harsh chemical peels or invasive cosmetic procedures, DMSO offers a gentle, non-invasive alternative that aligns with the growing demand for natural, sustainable skincare solutions. Over time, many users report that their skin looks brighter, more refreshed, and significantly more resilient to the effects of aging.

In a market saturated with synthetic products promising instant results, DMSO stands out as a simple yet powerful ally for those seeking a more natural path to youthful skin. By supporting the skin's health at a foundational level, it not only addresses the visible signs of aging but also promotes long-term vitality and radiance. Whether you're looking to reduce the appearance of existing wrinkles or maintain your skin's youthful glow, DMSO provides a versatile, effective tool for achieving your skincare goals.

Chapter 5

Internal Uses of DMSO and Controversies

DMSO's reputation as a natural remedy has been largely centered around topical applications, but a growing number of people are exploring its internal use. This side of DMSO—taken orally or injected—has stirred debate among both practitioners and researchers. While some suggest that internal DMSO use could offer immune support, reduced inflammation, and even relief from serious conditions, the controversy surrounding it is undeniable. Limited studies, anecdotal evidence, and varying safety concerns contribute to the skepticism, but understanding the science behind internal DMSO can help clarify where its potential benefits and risks lie.

The Science Behind Internal DMSO Usage

To understand DMSO's effects when taken internally, it helps to look at how it interacts with the body's systems. When ingested, DMSO is quickly absorbed and distributed throughout the body's tissues, crossing cell membranes with ease. Once inside the cells, DMSO is believed to reduce oxidative stress by scavenging free radicals, a process that could support overall cellular health. Because oxidative stress is implicated in a wide range of chronic diseases, from arthritis to neurodegenerative disorders, proponents of internal DMSO use believe it offers untapped benefits for those facing chronic inflammation and other health challenges.

However, the evidence supporting these claims remains sparse. Early research hinted at DMSO's anti-inflammatory potential and its ability to cross the blood-brain barrier, a unique trait that allows it to reach areas many drugs cannot. Yet, despite these promising properties, the body of rigorous clinical research on internal DMSO use remains limited. Most studies focus on topical applications, and while animal studies have shown some positive effects, the human data is less definitive. This gap in research is part of why internal DMSO use remains a controversial topic.

Potential Benefits for Immune Support

One of the compelling claims around internal DMSO use lies in its potential to fortify the immune system by reducing oxidative stress, a significant factor in both chronic disease and immune health. When oxidative stress occurs, free radicals, or unstable molecules, begin attacking healthy cells, leading to cell damage and aging. By neutralizing these free radicals, DMSO could help shield cells from harm and enhance immune resilience. This action is like providing an invisible layer of protection against the wear and tear that our cells face every day, which can accumulate over time and gradually weaken our immune defenses.

Inflammation and oxidative stress tend to work in tandem, often creating a feedback loop that's difficult to break. Inflammation heightens oxidative stress, which in turn promotes more inflammation, straining the immune system. DMSO, by reducing inflammation, may interrupt this cycle and free up the body's immune resources, allowing them to respond more effectively to threats. This could be particularly beneficial for those with chronic inflammatory conditions, where the immune system is under constant pressure.

Dr. Stanley Jacob, a leading DMSO researcher, was fascinated by this unique ability. He often noted that DMSO's anti-inflammatory properties might go beyond temporary relief and actually contribute to a more balanced immune response. While research remains in its early stages, there are numerous anecdotal reports from users who've noticed improvements in immune resilience. People with autoimmune conditions, for example, have shared stories of symptom reduction, though such cases are largely individual experiences rather than the result of controlled studies.

Some practitioners even suggest that pairing DMSO with well-known immune-supporting nutrients, such as vitamin C or zinc, may offer compounded benefits. Vitamin C, an antioxidant powerhouse, works alongside DMSO's neutralizing effects, potentially strengthening the immune system's response against common pathogens and reducing cell-damaging oxidative stress. Zinc, known for its immune-supportive properties, may help regulate immune function and promote cell repair. Together, these supplements could create a comprehensive approach to immune support when combined with DMSO.

However, it's essential to approach internal DMSO use with caution. Unlike topical applications, where DMSO's effects are generally localized, internal use circulates the compound throughout the body, raising the possibility of interactions with other substances. Because DMSO enhances absorption, it can amplify the effects of vitamins and other supplements, which could lead to unexpected reactions. Anyone considering this approach is advised to consult with a healthcare provider, ideally one familiar with alternative treatments, to determine a safe and effective combination. As the interest in DMSO's immune benefits grows, so does the importance of approaching its use thoughtfully and well-informed, balancing enthusiasm with evidence-based caution.

. . .

Safety and Risks of Internal DMSO Use

When it comes to internal use, safety is a major concern. One of the primary risks involves the purity of DMSO, as ingesting non-pharmaceutical-grade DMSO can introduce contaminants into the body. Only the highest purity forms of DMSO—typically labeled as "pharmaceutical grade" or "99.9% pure"—should ever be considered for internal use. Ingesting industrial or technical grade DMSO, which may contain impurities, poses a risk of adverse reactions and toxicity.

Proper dosing is also essential. Because DMSO is potent, even a small amount can have powerful effects. Diluting DMSO with distilled water is a standard practice for internal use, but exact dosages vary widely based on individual factors, such as body weight and health conditions. The lack of standardized dosing guidelines makes it even more important to consult a knowledgeable health practitioner before starting internal DMSO use. Medical consultation is crucial to assess potential interactions with existing medications and to ensure safe integration of DMSO into a treatment regimen.

DMSO in Alternative Cancer Treatment

Perhaps one of the most debated uses of DMSO is its application in alternative cancer treatments. Some proponents argue that DMSO can help alleviate cancer-related pain and improve quality of life for those undergoing treatment. There is a theory that DMSO, due to its anti-inflammatory and antioxidant properties, might slow the progression of certain types of cancer. Additionally, some alternative practitioners believe that DMSO can be used as a vehicle to enhance the effectiveness of other cancer treatments, such as intravenous vitamin C, by helping it penetrate tissues more effectively.

However, the use of DMSO in cancer treatment is met with significant caution and skepticism. The medical community remains largely unconvinced, citing the lack of substantial, peer-reviewed research to support these claims. Studies exploring DMSO's impact on cancer cells are limited and have not provided conclusive results. For this reason, anyone considering DMSO as part of a cancer treatment plan should approach it as a complementary option rather than a primary treatment and should consult their oncologist or a qualified health professional. While there are anecdotal success stories, current research does not support DMSO as a standalone cancer therapy.

Common Myths About Internal DMSO

Given its controversial nature, internal DMSO use has attracted its fair share of myths and misconceptions. One common myth is that DMSO is a cure-all solution, capable of addressing a wide range of ailments from arthritis to Alzheimer's with minimal effort. While DMSO does offer unique properties, it is by no means a miracle cure. Its effectiveness varies greatly depending on the individual, the condition being treated, and how it's used.

Another myth is that internal DMSO use is universally safe as long as the product is pure. In reality, even pure DMSO can have side effects, particularly when used improperly. For instance, consuming large doses without proper dilution can lead to digestive discomfort, headaches, and fatigue. Recognizing these risks and separating fact from fiction is essential for anyone considering internal DMSO.

The lack of research also gives rise to confusion and misinformation. Many proponents of internal DMSO use rely on personal anecdotes or unverified sources, which can obscure the facts. To ensure you're getting reliable information, look for guidance from reputable sources and consult with healthcare professionals familiar with DMSO. Distinguishing credible information from overblown claims is crucial, especially with a treatment as potent and complex as DMSO.

Chapter 6

Using DMSO for Athletic Performance

Athletic performance requires strength, resilience, and the ability to bounce back after intense physical demands. For many athletes, pain, soreness, and limited flexibility are part of the journey. However, as DMSO gains popularity, it's proving to be an effective, natural ally in recovery and performance enhancement. Whether you're a competitive athlete or simply someone who enjoys regular workouts, DMSO offers benefits that can help keep you in top form.

6.1 Pain Relief for Training and Competition

Athletes constantly push their bodies to the limit, training harder, running faster, and lifting heavier in pursuit of peak performance. But with that intense effort comes an inevitable downside: muscle soreness, joint stiffness, and occasional strains. These aches are often seen as the price of progress, but they can also slow recovery and hinder performance if not managed properly. Enter DMSO—a fast, effective solution for those looking to stay at the top of their game. Applied directly to the skin, DMSO helps athletes tackle pain and inflammation head-on, offering relief that goes beyond the surface.

For athletes dealing with muscle strain or post-workout soreness, DMSO is a powerful ally. Its anti-inflammatory properties target swelling in muscles and joints, reducing pressure on nerve endings and alleviating discomfort. This means quicker recovery times and the ability to maintain consistent training without being derailed by lingering pain. Whether it's the result of a grueling weightlifting session or a high-impact cardio workout, DMSO can help soothe overworked muscles, keeping athletes in the game longer and with less downtime.

Many athletes have discovered the benefits of applying DMSO immediately after intense physical activity. Post-workout application is especially valuable after high-stress events such as marathons, competitive matches, or heavy training sessions, where the body is pushed to its limits. By using DMSO shortly after exercise, athletes can address soreness before it escalates, preventing stiffness and reducing the buildup of lactic acid—a key factor behind muscle fatigue and soreness. Lactic acid forms when the body produces energy anaerobically during intense exercise, leading to that familiar post-workout burn. DMSO's unique ability to enhance circulation and clear metabolic waste helps mitigate this effect, offering quicker relief and faster recovery.

To maximize its benefits and avoid potential issues, athletes typically dilute DMSO before application, especially if they're new to using it or treating sensitive areas. A common method involves mixing it with distilled water or aloe vera gel to create a solution that's both effective and gentle on the skin. Application is straightforward: using clean hands, a cotton cloth, or a soft applicator, athletes gently dab the DMSO onto the affected areas, ensuring even coverage without excessive rubbing. It's crucial to let the solution fully absorb before touching other parts of the body or putting on clothing, as DMSO can carry other substances through the skin—a feature that's both a strength and a caution.

For those serious about optimizing their recovery, consistency is key. Integrating DMSO into a post-workout routine can significantly reduce downtime between training sessions. Athletes who use DMSO regularly report less muscle fatigue, improved mobility, and an overall sense of readiness for their next challenge. Over time, this can lead to better performance and reduced risk of overuse injuries, allowing athletes to train smarter and recover faster.

6.2 Increasing Flexibility and Joint Mobility

Flexibility and joint mobility are the unsung heroes of

athletic performance. Whether you're a runner pounding the pavement, a cyclist conquering hills, or a weightlifter chasing new personal records, the ability to move freely and without pain is critical. Even disciplines like yoga, which prioritize fluid movement and controlled stretches, rely heavily on healthy, supple joints. DMSO's unique ability to penetrate deeply into tissues and joint capsules makes it a powerful ally for athletes seeking to enhance flexibility and maintain peak mobility.

One of the standout features of DMSO is its capacity to reduce stiffness in joints, allowing for smoother, more fluid movement. Athletes who struggle with restricted mobility in high-use areas like the knees, elbows, or shoulders often turn to DMSO as a natural solution. By reaching deep into the joint capsule, DMSO helps to alleviate inflammation and lubricate the joint, making it easier to achieve a full range of motion. This is particularly beneficial for those recovering from joint injuries, where stiffness can linger long after the initial injury has healed, limiting performance and increasing the risk of reinjury.

To maximize the benefits of DMSO for joint mobility, many athletes incorporate it into their pre-workout routine. Applying a diluted DMSO solution to key joints before stretching exercises can help warm up the tissues, making muscles and joints more pliable. This combination of DMSO and stretching not only enhances flexibility but also ensures that stretches are performed more safely, reducing the risk of strains or tears. For athletes in recovery, this practice is invaluable. It helps maintain range of motion and combats the stiffness that often accompanies prolonged periods of rest or immobilization.

DMSO's benefits extend beyond warm-ups. Many athletes also apply it post-game or after intense practices to soothe joints that have been subjected to heavy strain. A light application to areas like the hips, shoulders, or ankles can help reduce inflammation and ease discomfort, speeding up recovery and preparing the body for the next session. This dual approach—using DMSO both before and after activity—provides comprehensive support, helping athletes maintain their mobility even under the rigorous demands of daily training and competition.

Chapter 7

Beyond Pain – DMSO for Everyday Wellness

DMSO is often celebrated for its pain-relieving properties, but its potential extends far beyond that. When used thoughtfully, it becomes a versatile addition to an everyday wellness routine, supporting physical and mental health. In this chapter, we'll explore how DMSO can be used to manage stress, improve circulation, enhance sleep quality, boost cognitive clarity, and create a sustainable wellness plan.

7.1 Managing Stress with DMSO

Stress is often thought of as a mental or emotional burden, but its impact on the body is just as profound. It creeps into your muscles, tightening your neck, stiffening your shoulders, and leaving your lower back in knots. Over time, this physical tension can snowball, contributing to headaches, fatigue, and even chronic pain. This is where DMSO can play a transformative role. Known for its anti-inflammatory and muscle-relaxing properties, DMSO offers a natural, effective way to release physical stress and bring your body back to a state of ease.

When stress-induced tension builds up, DMSO can be applied directly to the problem areas—whether it's the tight bands of muscle across your shoulders, the base of your neck, or that persistent ache in your lower back. As it penetrates the skin, DMSO works to reduce inflammation and relax muscle fibers, alleviating the pressure and discomfort caused by stress. This isn't just surface-level relief; DMSO targets the underlying inflammation and tension that keep your muscles locked up, offering a deeper, more lasting sense of relaxation.

To take things a step further, many people incorporate DMSO into their relaxation rituals. Applying DMSO to tension points, followed by a gentle massage, can amplify its benefits. The act of massaging not only helps distribute the DMSO more evenly but also stimulates circulation, enhancing its ability to reach deeper tissues. For an even more soothing experience, you can apply a warm compress over the treated area after applying DMSO. The heat encourages muscle relaxation, deepens the penetration of DMSO, and provides an immediate calming sensation.

For those who practice mindfulness or meditation, DMSO can be a powerful companion. Before settling into a meditation session, try applying a small amount of DMSO to your temples, wrists, or the back of your neck.

Its calming effect can help release the lingering physical tension that often distracts from mental focus, allowing you to sink more deeply into your practice. The sensation of relief that DMSO provides can serve as a physical anchor, grounding your body and enhancing your sense of presence.

7.2 Improving Circulation and Cardiovascular Health

DMSO's ability to enhance circulation is yet another remarkable benefit, particularly for those aiming to boost their cardiovascular health. Healthy circulation plays a pivotal role in overall well-being, ensuring that oxygen and nutrients are efficiently delivered to cells while waste products are promptly removed. When circulation falters, energy levels can plummet, extremities may feel cold or numb, and muscle cramps or aches can become all too common. DMSO, with its unique ability to relax blood vessels, offers a natural way to support and improve blood flow, providing both immediate relief and long-term benefits.

Poor circulation often manifests as cold hands and feet, muscle stiffness, or cramps—especially in the legs. These symptoms can be frustrating and even debilitating, limiting mobility and reducing quality of life. DMSO works by relaxing the smooth muscles within blood vessel walls, promoting vasodilation and allowing blood to flow more freely. This makes it particularly useful for individuals who experience cramping, cold extremities, or other circulation-related discomforts. Unlike many topical solutions that provide only surface-level relief, DMSO penetrates deeply, addressing the root causes of these issues by improving blood flow where it's needed most.

For targeted circulation support, DMSO can be applied to areas where blood flow tends to be naturally limited or where discomfort occurs. For example, applying DMSO to the calves can help alleviate painful leg cramps, which are often caused by restricted circulation or overexertion. Similarly, massaging a diluted DMSO solution into the hands or feet can bring immediate warmth and increased mobility to these often-affected extremities, making it a valuable tool for those who struggle with poor peripheral circulation.

To maximize its benefits, many users incorporate DMSO into their daily cardiovascular routines. Applying DMSO after activities like brisk walking, light stretching, or yoga can amplify its effects. These movements naturally promote blood flow, and the addition of DMSO helps sustain and enhance this circulation even after the activity has ended. This combination not only supports cardiovascular health but also boosts overall vitality, leaving you feeling more energized and less prone to the sluggishness that poor circulation can cause.

7.3 Sleep Support and Relaxation

A restful night's sleep can feel elusive when discomfort or tension keeps you tossing and turning. Whether it's muscle soreness from the day's activities or the persistent ache of chronic pain, these physical barriers to sleep can leave you feeling drained before the new day even begins. This is where DMSO steps in as a natural solution, offering not just pain relief but a pathway to deeper, more restorative rest.

DMSO's dual action of alleviating pain and relaxing tense muscles makes it an ideal addition to your bedtime routine. By targeting areas of discomfort—whether it's the lower back, shoulders, or legs—DMSO helps reduce the physical stress that can prevent you from falling asleep. Its deep-penetrating properties work quickly to calm inflamed tissues, allowing your body to transition more smoothly into a state of relaxation. This not only helps you fall asleep faster but also improves the quality of your sleep, reducing those frequent awakenings caused by lingering pain or stiffness.

Incorporating DMSO into your nightly ritual doesn't have to be complicated. A simple yet effective approach is to apply a diluted solution to sore or tight areas about 20–30 minutes before bed. For an added layer of relaxation, consider blending DMSO with a few drops of lavender or chamomile essential oil. These natural scents are known for their calming properties and can help signal to your mind and body that it's time to unwind. The combination of DMSO's muscle-relaxing effects and the soothing aroma creates a sensory experience that prepares you for restful sleep.

Beyond physical relief, the act of applying DMSO can become a mindful practice, helping to establish a sense of routine and calm before bed. As you gently massage the solution into your skin, focus on your breathing, letting each exhale release the tension of the day. This intentional winding down, paired with other sleep-promoting habits such as dimming the lights, avoiding screens, and practicing gratitude or meditation, creates an environment conducive to deep, uninterrupted sleep.

7.4 DMSO for Cognitive Clarity

Cognitive clarity and focus are crucial in today's demanding world, yet many people experience mental fog and fatigue, whether from stress, lack of sleep, or health issues. Although primarily known for its physical benefits, DMSO's role in reducing inflammation and oxidative stress may indirectly support mental clarity, giving it potential as a cognitive aid.

For those who experience brain fog, adding DMSO to a daily routine may help improve focus over time. Although DMSO is not a stimulant, its ability to reduce inflammation can have a refreshing effect on cognitive energy, potentially making it easier to concentrate. Some users incorporate DMSO by applying a diluted amount to pulse points or areas like the back of the neck, where it may relieve tension that contributes to mental fatigue. Combined with other cognitive-supportive practices, such as hydration, regular breaks, and mental exercises, DMSO can be a subtle yet powerful addition to a mental clarity regimen.

7.5 Creating a Long-Term DMSO Wellness Plan

Incorporating DMSO into your wellness routine isn't just about short-term relief; it's about building a sustainable, long-term plan that aligns with your health goals. Thoughtful planning and realistic expectations are key to getting the most out of this powerful natural remedy. Whether you're aiming to ease joint stiffness, improve sleep quality, enhance flexibility, or reduce stress, setting clear, measurable goals helps guide your journey and track your progress effectively.

Start by identifying the areas of your life where you'd like to see improvement. For instance, if joint stiffness has been holding you back, your goal might be to regain mobility and comfort through consistent DMSO application. Similarly, if stress manifests as muscle tension or poor sleep, you can focus on using DMSO to target those specific challenges. Clear goals not only provide direction but also help you stay motivated as you begin to notice gradual improvements.

When integrating DMSO into your daily routine, gradual implementation is essential. Begin with small, manageable applications and pay close attention to how your body responds. For new users, this might mean starting with a diluted solution applied once a day to a specific area, such as the lower back or knees. As your body becomes accustomed to DMSO, you can slowly increase the frequency or expand its use to other areas as needed. The key is to listen to your body and adjust accordingly, ensuring that your routine remains both effective and comfortable.

For long-term success, creating a structured wellness plan can help you stay consistent. This could involve setting a weekly or monthly schedule that aligns with your lifestyle. For example, you might apply DMSO after workouts to support recovery or before bed to enhance relaxation and sleep. Over time, this routine becomes second nature, seamlessly fitting into your broader wellness strategy.

Tracking your progress is another valuable tool in your long-term plan. Maintaining a simple journal or log of your DMSO applications allows you to monitor its effects and make informed adjustments. Record details such as the concentration used, the area of application, and any noticeable changes in symptoms, mood, energy levels, or overall well-being. This not only provides a clear picture of your progress but also helps identify patterns or areas where further adjustments might be beneficial.

Chapter 8

Advanced Tips and FAQs for Mastering DMSO Use

By now, you have a solid understanding of DMSO's basics and its potential applications. This final chapter is designed for those ready to take their DMSO use to the next level. Here, we'll explore advanced application techniques, address common issues, answer frequently asked questions, and guide you in integrating DMSO into a holistic health regimen. Whether you're looking to optimize your approach or dive into the finer points of DMSO, this chapter has you covered.

8.1 Advanced Application Techniques

As versatile as DMSO is, knowing a few advanced techniques can help you maximize its benefits for specific issues. One powerful strategy involves layering DMSO with other natural remedies. For example, combining DMSO with magnesium oil can provide a dual-action solution for muscle cramps, targeting both pain and tension. Other users find success layering DMSO with herbal salves or essential oils, using it as a carrier to enhance absorption and effectiveness. Just remember to test small areas first to ensure compatibility.

Creating your own DMSO blends is another advanced technique. Some users mix DMSO with soothing agents like aloe vera or coconut oil, creating custom solutions for sensitive skin. For particular issues—such as deep muscle pain—adding a few drops of essential oils like peppermint or eucalyptus to DMSO can bring targeted relief. Just be cautious with essential oils, as they can be potent; a small amount goes a long way.

For hard-to-reach areas or sensitive spots, try using DMSO in gel form. Gels are easier to control and can adhere better to the skin without dripping, making them perfect for applications on the neck, spine, or specific joint areas. This method allows for precision and reduces the risk of unintended transfer to other parts of the body.

8.2 Troubleshooting Common Issues

As with any powerful compound, using DMSO comes with a learning curve. Skin irritation is one of the most common issues new users face. If irritation occurs, consider diluting your DMSO solution further, and always apply it to clean, dry skin to avoid contamination.

Applying a small amount of a soothing agent like aloe vera afterward can help calm any initial discomfort.

Adjusting your dosage is another part of the DMSO journey. While it's natural to start with low doses, some users find they need to gradually increase or fine-tune the amount for optimal results. Let your body's feedback guide you. If you experience mild side effects—like a headache or slight fatigue—this may be your body's way of signaling that it needs more time to adjust. Managing side effects is often as simple as lowering the dose temporarily or spacing out applications.

Finally, be mindful of interactions with other topicals. Avoid applying DMSO immediately after using lotions or other skincare products, as it can enhance their absorption in unintended ways. Clear skin creates the cleanest, safest experience with DMSO.

8.3 Incorporating DMSO into Other Health Practices

DMSO's versatility makes it an invaluable addition to a variety of health practices, enhancing the effectiveness of both physical and lifestyle-based wellness routines. Its unique properties allow it to synergize with other treatments, amplifying their benefits and helping users achieve better, more sustainable outcomes. Whether you're focusing on physical therapy, dietary changes, or holistic detox strategies, DMSO can fit seamlessly into your health plan.

In the realm of physical therapy, DMSO serves as a powerful ally. Applied to sore or tense areas before a session, it can help reduce inflammation and ease muscle stiffness, making it easier to engage in therapeutic exercises. For those recovering from injuries or managing chronic conditions like arthritis, this can be a game-changer. By increasing joint mobility and alleviating pain, DMSO allows patients to perform stretches and movements more effectively, maximizing the benefits of each session. Massage therapy also pairs well with DMSO; when applied beforehand, it enhances the therapist's ability to work deeper into the tissues, leading to greater muscle relaxation and improved circulation.

DMSO's benefits extend beyond physical treatments to include dietary and detoxification practices. Pairing DMSO with an anti-inflammatory diet can create a compounding effect, tackling inflammation from multiple angles. Foods rich in omega-3 fatty acids, antioxidants, and other anti-inflammatory compounds work in harmony with DMSO's cellular-level action, helping to reduce systemic inflammation more effectively. Similarly, incorporating DMSO into a detox routine can enhance the body's natural toxin elimination processes. DMSO's ability to penetrate tissues deeply may assist in flushing out accumulated toxins, particularly when paired with increased hydration and a nutrient-dense diet.

8.4 Resources for Continued Learning

The journey with DMSO doesn't end with this book. As a powerful and multifaceted compound, its potential continues to unfold with ongoing research and evolving best practices. Staying informed is essential to ensure you're making the most of DMSO's benefits while using it safely and effectively. Fortunately, there are plenty of resources available to help you deepen your understanding and keep up with the latest developments.

For those who prefer in-depth exploration, books and articles by respected experts in the field are a great starting point. Works by pioneers like Dr. Stanley Jacob, often referred to as the "father of DMSO research," offer valuable historical and scientific context. These resources delve into advanced applications, provide case studies, and offer practical advice based on decades of research and clinical experience. Additionally, newer publications by alternative health practitioners and scientific researchers provide updated perspectives on DMSO's role in modern wellness routines.

Online resources are another excellent way to stay current. Websites dedicated to natural health and alternative medicine frequently publish updates on DMSO, including summaries of new studies, expert interviews, and user testimonials. Scientific research databases and journals are also worth exploring for those interested in the technical details of how DMSO works and its expanding list of potential applications.

Equally valuable is the opportunity to connect with other DMSO users. Joining online forums, social media groups, or communities focused on alternative treatments can provide a wealth of practical knowledge. These platforms allow users to share their experiences, offer tips, and troubleshoot common challenges. Whether you're curious about how others incorporate DMSO into their routines or want to explore new uses for specific health concerns, these communities offer a supportive and informative environment. Hearing firsthand accounts from people who have successfully used DMSO can be both inspiring and reassuring, especially for newcomers.

As research on DMSO continues, staying engaged with the latest findings empowers you to make informed decisions and discover innovative ways to enhance your health journey. By leveraging these resources, you can deepen your knowledge, refine your techniques, and remain at the forefront of DMSO's evolving story. The more you learn, the more confident and effective you'll become in integrating this remarkable compound into your long-term wellness strategy.

Epilogue

DMSO is a revolution in natural health. This powerful, unassuming molecule has the potential to redefine how you approach pain, healing, and wellness as a whole. Imagine finally breaking free from chronic pain that's haunted you for years. Picture rejuvenated, glowing skin, faster recovery after intense workouts, and true relief that comes from addressing issues at their very core. DMSO does all of this and more. Unlike conventional treatments that only skim the surface, DMSO goes deep, working on a cellular level to bring lasting change. This isn't about quick fixes; it's about solutions that actually work and keep working.

DMSO's true power lies in its versatility. It's not just for one problem, one symptom, or one area. It adapts to a range of needs, fitting seamlessly into different parts of your life. You can use it to calm aching joints, improve flexibility, clear up skin, reduce scars, and even enhance your sleep quality. It's like having an all-in-one wellness tool that responds to your specific needs, helping you live and feel your best in every aspect. And with DMSO, it's not about temporary relief—it's about giving you the tools to create real, sustainable change.

Through this guide, you've learned that DMSO isn't just another product. It's a complete approach to health, offering benefits for daily wellness, targeted healing, and even peak performance for athletes. DMSO goes beyond basic support; it optimizes. It empowers you to approach your health from a place of knowledge, confidence, and genuine self-care. It's there when you need it, whether for chronic aches, sudden flare-ups, or a holistic boost to your wellness routine.

But the impact of DMSO doesn't end with simply using it. By taking the time to understand its mechanisms and applying it thoughtfully, you've gained a powerful skill set that puts you in control. You know how to make DMSO work for you, and that means more than just applying a product—it means approaching each day with the confidence that you have a tool for immediate relief and gradual, lasting wellness. DMSO is now part of your journey, giving you reliable, effective support on your terms.

And this isn't just another supplement—it's a full-bodied approach to wellness that respects your body's own healing processes. DMSO has become part of a sustainable health path, one that aligns with the way you want to feel: vibrant, pain-free, and empowered. You're not just adding another remedy; you're choosing a future with fewer limitations, greater resilience, and an approach that's as natural as it is effective.

With DMSO by your side, you're stepping into a future of better health, less pain, and a renewed sense of well-being. This journey isn't just about what DMSO can do for you today; it's about creating a foundation for a life lived fully—one that embraces health not as a fleeting goal, but as a lifestyle. Embrace DMSO as your trusted companion on this path to lasting health, and know that with every step, you're building a stronger, healthier, more empowered version of yourself.

DMSO Usage Checklist

Preparation & Precautions

- ☐ **Use Only High-Purity DMSO**: Always choose pharmaceutical-grade (99.9% pure) DMSO to avoid impurities that could cause adverse reactions.
- ☐ **Dilute for Initial Use**: Start with a diluted solution (e.g., 70% DMSO with 30% distilled water) to test sensitivity, especially for sensitive skin or new users.
- ☐ **Test a Small Area First**: Apply a small amount on a patch of skin (such as your forearm) and wait 24 hours to check for any irritation or adverse reactions.
- ☐ **Work with Clean, Dry Skin**: Ensure the area is thoroughly cleansed and dried

before application to prevent DMSO from carrying in dirt or other substances.
- ☐ **Store Properly**: Keep DMSO in a cool, dark place, ideally in a glass container, as DMSO can degrade certain plastics.

Mixing & Application Techniques

- ☐ **Use Distilled Water or Aloe Vera for Dilution**: For sensitive applications or areas, dilute DMSO with distilled water or aloe vera to reduce potency.
- ☐ **Avoid Mixing with Lotions or Other Topicals**: Apply only to bare skin to avoid unintended absorption of other substances.
- ☐ **Apply with Non-Contaminating Tools**: Use clean, disposable cotton balls or applicators; if using hands, ensure they are washed thoroughly.
- ☐ **Wear Gloves When Needed**: Latex or nitrile gloves are recommended, especially for high-concentration solutions or repeated applications.

Application Dos & Don'ts

- ☐ **DO Let DMSO Air Dry**: Allow it to

dry naturally without covering the area for maximum absorption.
- ☐ **DO Start with Shorter Exposure Times**: Limit initial applications to 20-30 minutes before rinsing off, and extend time gradually as comfort allows.
- ☐ **DON'T Apply DMSO to Open Wounds**: Avoid using it on open cuts or broken skin, as this can cause irritation or stinging.
- ☐ **DON'T Combine DMSO with Harsh or Strong Chemicals**: Ensure that any additional products used on the skin are mild, as DMSO can intensify their effects.

Frequency & Routine

- ☐ **Establish a Safe Routine**: Start with once-daily applications and assess how your body responds. Increase frequency gradually if needed and tolerated well.
- ☐ **Track Results and Adjust as Needed**: Keep a log of DMSO applications and any noticeable effects, adjusting dosage or frequency based on observed results.
- ☐ **Rest and Monitor for Side Effects**: Watch for any signs of irritation or discomfort. If any occur, dilute the solution further or reduce the frequency of applications.

Safe Mixing, Storing, and Application

Mixing Your DMSO Solution

☐ **Decide on Your Desired Concentration**:

For 60%: Mix 6 parts DMSO with 4 parts distilled water or aloe vera.

For 70%: Mix 7 parts DMSO with 3 parts distilled water or aloe vera.

For 80%: Mix 8 parts DMSO with 2 parts distilled water or aloe vera.

☐ **Use Distilled Water** (or Aloe Vera Gel)**:**

Distilled water is recommended because it's free from minerals or contaminants that may react with DMSO.

For sensitive applications, mixing with aloe vera gel can create a gentler solution while still maintaining effectiveness.

Safe Mixing, Storing, and Application

☐ **Mix in a Clean, Glass Container**:

DMSO can degrade certain plastics, so use glass whenever possible.

Measure carefully using a dropper, syringe, or graduated measuring cup to maintain accurate concentrations.

Storing Your DMSO Solution

☐ **Store in a Dark, Cool Place**:

Keep your DMSO solution away from direct sunlight, ideally in an amber or blue glass bottle to protect it from light.

Room temperature is usually fine, but some prefer refrigeration for long-term storage.

☐ **Label with Concentration and Date**:

Clearly label each bottle with the concentration (e.g., "70% DMSO") and the date it was mixed.

Discard and mix a new solution if you notice cloudiness or particles, which can indicate contamination.

Topical Application Steps

☐ **Clean and Dry Skin**:

Wash the area with mild soap and water, then let it dry completely before application.

Avoid any lotions or other products on the skin before using DMSO.

Safe Mixing, Storing, and Application

☐ **Apply with a Cotton Ball or Applicator**:

Using clean, disposable cotton balls or a soft cloth is best. Apply sparingly and avoid drenching the area.

If you're using a higher concentration (80% or more), apply with gloves to protect your hands.

☐ **Let DMSO Air Dry**:

Leave the applied DMSO uncovered to dry naturally for maximum absorption.

Wait at least 20-30 minutes before rinsing or covering the area if necessary.

☐ **Monitor Skin for Irritation**:

If you experience tingling, itching, or redness, try diluting your solution further or reducing application frequency.

Internal Dosing Guidelines

☐ **Start with a Low Dose**:

For beginners, try a very small dose, such as 1-2 drops of 50% diluted DMSO mixed in 6-8 oz. of distilled water or juice.

Gradually increase if well-tolerated, but proceed with caution.

☐ **Mix with Distilled Water or Juice**:

Distilled Water: Preferred for purity; DMSO

Safe Mixing, Storing, and Application

dissolves easily in distilled water, minimizing the risk of contaminants.

Juice: Some find that mixing with a mild juice (such as aloe vera or cranberry) improves taste and palatability.

☐ **Take by Dropperful, Not by Full Dropper**:

Start with a few drops (up to a quarter dropperful) and observe how your body responds. Increase only as tolerated.

Avoid full droppers without guidance; a small dose is effective and safer to start.

☐ **Follow with Plain Water**:

After taking DMSO, drink a full glass of water to help with absorption and dilute any lingering taste.

Monitor for any adverse reactions, and if you experience stomach discomfort, lower the dose or stop and consult a professional.

Final Tips for Safe and Effective Use

☐ **Use DMSO Sparingly and Increase Slowly**:

Less is more; begin with small amounts and gradually increase, allowing your body to adjust.

Topical users can start with once-daily applications and observe results before increasing frequency.

☐ **Consult a Healthcare Provider for Internal Use**:

Safe Mixing, Storing, and Application

Internal dosing is potent and should be approached with care. Discuss with a healthcare professional, especially if combining with other supplements or medications.

www.ingramcontent.com/pod-product-compliance
Lightning Source LLC
Chambersburg PA
CBHW052334220526
45472CB00001B/411